Healing The Broken Pieces Of My Life And Yours

A Transformative Journey Into Healing

France is a transformational author, speaker, Reiki healer and mentor. She facilitates workshops with a mission to assist in the uncovering and healing of the broken pieces in your life.

Connect with her at:
www.FranceBarringer.com
and claim your free one hour breakthrough session today!

France Barringer

CONTENTS

PREFACE

As you are reading these words in this very moment, you may not consciously realize it, but your higher self has led you to these pages. You may call it your inner wisdom, intuition, spirit, guidance, or even providence. But the real beauty is that you have listened to the subtle whispers that have brought you here. You have acknowledged the You that on some level, desires to be heard, understood, seen, and subsequently, healed and empowered.

In order to walk the path of growth, healing, and completeness with the past, we need someone we can trust to lead us through the present—because we can't do this alone. We need a teacher that can take our hand and be human with us.

The greatest of teachers don't say "follow me" but rather "I'll go first". Their courage to step into the unknown and hold a torch to illuminate our path is a gift beyond measure. Should you be so fortunate to meet such a teacher, you will have been one of the very few to have this privilege. Prepare to be one of the fortunate few.

France Barringer is much more than the author of this book. She is that once-in-a lifetime teacher that has walked the path and is now reaching out her hand, inviting you to take the journey that you've been reluctant to go on your entire life, until now.

Many authors write their life story, and as the reader, sometimes you feel like you are a detached, outside observer of their life. However, France's life story will awaken *your* story. The breadth, richness, and depth of France's emotions in her life are not unique to her—they are emotions that we *all* have felt on some level to varying degrees. Yet, so many of us have lacked the love, support, and compassion needed to unlock the vault of our inner most feelings that have been yearning to be noticed. But now, your imperfections are safe to emerge and come out in the open as France stands in hers with an honesty that is so refreshing and inspiring.

The true bravery of this book is the masterful way in which France shares her story with vulnerability and transparency that is to be admired. With organic and unfiltered emotions, France gets to the core of human emotion in a way that will grip you, push you to the edge, and evoke emotions rooted so deep within you that have been unconsciously running your life.

This book will uproot everything you have suppressed and ignored just to survive. France's story goes way beyond survival, and into the triumph of learning how to truly live by overcoming your biggest fears. This is an invitation for you to stop surviving, and start living life to the fullest.

It takes a wise soul to know that the thing that scares us the most is the thing that we're most meant to be doing. In this book, you will not only see how France faced her biggest fears head on by writing her story, but you will come to understand that her Divine purpose is to help you find yours.

And as you read France's story, you might think to yourself, "If France can overcome everything she did and find inner peace, it's time for me to look at myself and start living the life I was meant to live!"

As a testament to the authentic nature of this book, France asked me, her youngest son, to write this preface. As unconventional as this might be, it illustrates that time and again, she shows us the beauty of coloring outside the lines, challenging conformity, and how to find our own unique voice in a sea of humanity.

As you will discover, I have shared in much of my Mom's journey. Yet, as I read her book, it felt as though I was hearing everything for the first time. With a purity and innocence that is so hard to find in today's world, I'm confident in saying that as you read this book, you will feel like you can relate to her. You will feel connected. You will feel emotions down to your bones. You will feel like you are not alone on your journey. You will feel a sense of hope, release, freedom, and excitement for what's ahead.

As her proud son, it has been a privilege to see my Mom evolve into a teacher beyond my life, and that of humanity. And what I love most about this book is that France inspires in two ways.

1) By her example and how she's overcome adversity in ways that are nothing short of heroic.

2) By giving you very practical tools so that you can overcome *your* fears on the path to *your* healing.

Many times, people overcome great odds and leave us inspired, but don't share *how* we can do this in *our* lives. However, should you choose to transform your life, France has provided a guide book that will help you to face your biggest challenges and experience the healing, forgiveness, and ultimately, self love that waits for you on the other side. For once you can love yourself, love will flow to others in ways that are natural to the human spirit, not to the human mind.

I have often heard people say that it is a miracle that my Mom turned out to be so vibrant and full of life given the challenges of her life. Yet, the real miracle is the one that lives inside each of us, ready to be awakened from its life-long slumber. This book will be your soul's alarm clock.

As a singer/songwriter, I have written many original songs. But there is one in particular that holds a special place in my heart called "Angel On The Ground" that I wrote for my Mom. Once you read this book, you will experience how she can be an angel in *your* life. I believe Angels come in many forms. This one has come in the form of my mother.

Honoring you on your courageous journey,
Tiamo De Vettori

Testimonials

As a Marriage and Family Therapist, I see the ongoing struggles of my clients when attempting to heal from past traumas/experiences and the effects on their current life situations and relationships. I too, like anyone else, am consistently searching for ways of healing my own traumas so I can assist others in healing theirs. Healing the Broken Pieces is a book I personally and professionally recommend to anyone who is struggling to heal their past in order to have a more peaceful present and successful future. France articulately, and vulnerably, shared her own life challenges and struggles and how she overcame them. France is one of those daring souls whose courage and openness is something only a select few would willingly create. The techniques and exercises in the healing guidebook were created to heal herself and all those she has come in contact with, including myself. France is not only a talented writer she is an experienced survivor, a wayshower, soul searcher and friend to all. If you are ready to take a leap in healing the broken pieces of your life, then you are ready to go on the journey of her life story and the steps she shares in her healing guidebook "Healing the Broken Pieces of my Life and Yours." I warn you, be prepared to cry, laugh, love and most of all HEAL."

Besan Hanna, Bilingual Arabic/English Marriage and Family Therapist

Spiritual Warrior, France Barringer, provokes with her two book series, "Healing the Broken Pieces of my Life" and her follow-up workbook, "Healing the Broken Pieces of my Life and Yours." Each is a masterpiece in its own right but together they are simply brilliant. A powerful tribute to life, and a spirit that cannot be broken, these books will most likely bring you to tears. Following France through her personal rabbit hole into spiritual maturation and the life that seemed to weave around her was heart-wrenching but true to form. She never failed to make me laugh, cry, and ponder with each riveting turn. This series is a rousing tribute to the pivotal role of choice and the importance of listening to one's heart. It is a must read for anyone who is serious about breaking the bonds that chain them and leaves in exchange the healing emotions of wonder, joy, compassion and hope. France truly is a light in this world and her books are a testament to the transformation that can occur. They have the power to change your life!

Chelsa Michelsen, M.S., Intuitive Astrologer

Do you feel broken inside?

How to discover, embrace, transform and empower yourself through the broken pieces of your life.

In her "can't put it down" life story, **Healing The Broken Pieces of My Life**, companion of this healing guidebook, after recalling tragic events from her past, the author discovers that *unhealed* emotions are still part of her. As she unravels the gift in each broken piece of her life she gains the freedom to live her life with joy, renewal, peace and strength.

This healing guidebook offers you an opportunity to find your own way towards the freedom and peace that you utterly deserve by

- Discovering unhealed emotions and how they affect your body
- Identifying your deepest emotional triggers and how to heal them
- Raising your level of consciousness
- Connecting and listening to your mind, body and soul
- Living an empowering life

You don't have to remain broken . . . *Whole is what you are meant to be.*

Introduction to Healing your Broken Pieces

"There can be no greater tragedy than living an unexamined life" Plato wrote that and he was right.

Do you wonder why you feel depressed or tired all the time? Why you procrastinate, drink or eat too much? Why you can't be in a good relationship or find a good career? Do you feel victimized by the world around you or are you angry and frustrated most of the time?

Although I examined my life, I was not finding the solutions to my problems until…I examined my "self" which created the life that I am now living. Here is my own quote: *"There can be no greater tragedy than living an unexamined self"* and that became a prerequisite to understanding the meaning of my life.

Even if I had a greater understanding of my feelings and behaviors through the help of therapy, spiritual teachings and self-help books, I had not yet reached the *Holy Grail*. I was yearning for greater knowledge to shift my "self" and live an empowered life as oppose to a victimized life.

What is a victimized life? It's when you live a life full of dramas involving your family, work situations, friends, and relationships. It's when you are living your life as a victim and you are suffering most of the time. Of course my first recollection of the world was at age two and set the stage of what was to unfold. I was going to live in a very scary and unfair world.

Although I was a victim, I must say that I never felt helpless as I always found a solution to my problems. So, for the sake of clarification, I was an "empowered victim." There is also another type of victim, one who is helpless. Sounds familiar? Welcome to *Healing The Broken Pieces Of My Life and Yours*. This guidebook will hopefully become your *Holy Grail* and your salvation.

How? By becoming whole. Wholeness comes in 3 parts: Mind, body and soul. Integrating those 3 aspects of your being will make you complete. I was fragmented and I knew it. What I didn't know was that by looking at my broken pieces I would become whole and free from suffering. Notice that I didn't say from pain. As long as I remain alive, I believe I will experience pain. I may grieve the loss of someone close to me and will feel the pain, but suffering is different. Suffering keeps one stuck in the pain.

Because I was *victimized* most of my life, I often blamed the circumstances and the people that caused me to suffer. Although I kept changing my life's conditions and surrounded myself with different people, I subconsciously, without my awareness recreated patterns that caused me to suffer.

I congratulate you in making the right choice. Ahead of you is a journey of self-healing, wholeness, hope, freedom, and opportunities for a new life but most of all, a journey of nothing less than a miracle discovering "YOU" in mind, body and soul.

Welcome to your broken pieces. This is your sacred guidebook and journey!

Warning: After completing and practicing all of the steps in this guidebook, you will never feel like a victim again. There is a payoff in being a victim, which is very hard for the ego to let go. Why? It's because the ego finds justification and gratification in blaming other people for the way that you feel and keep you stuck in your life drama. You also don't have to be accountable and take responsibility for the way that you feel. You won't get to hear the "Oh poor you," "How horrible your life has been!" or "You are such a survivor!" Although these statements may be true, to continue to blame others will never empower you. My intention is not to diminish what has happened to you. It was wrong to be violated either physically, verbally, mentally or spiritually and yes...you were a victim! Even if you may have been a victim, the way out of victimhood is not to remain in that role but to have the courage to find another way.

My way is not the only way but it is a way that works. It worked for me and it can work for you. Give it a try. What do you have to lose? A victimized life… is what you will lose.

You will be in the driver seat, which means that you will be the one in charge of your own feelings and emotions. And you will acquire freedom by really letting go of the past events that have haunted you all of those years. You will be able to redesign your life the way you choose to live it and no longer be at the mercy of your circumstances… no matter what they are. You can change them. It begins with your decision today to create a better way of living your life, away from suffering. Are you ready?

First, let's look at the different ways that we handle our feelings.

Because we don't like to suffer, we often *suppress* the feelings that we experience. In other words, we resist feeling our emotions. We push them down, thinking that they will go away although they never do. The resistance inflicted upon ourselves creates a tremendous amount of pressure that is often felt in the physical body as a form of back or neck problems and many other physical conditions. The emotional body also feels this resistance through a form of anxiety, depression, mood swings and many other emotional conditions.

Unconsciously, the mind uses different mechanisms to keep these feelings away from our awareness. *Denial* is a very favorite method used by the mind to block the undesired feelings. We deny the existence of the painful feelings and we may try to escape them through the use of drugs, alcohol, food, sex or work.

Another favorite method used by the mind, is *projection*. We project into the world and the people around us the feelings that we *repress*. So, instead of feeling them, we experience the feelings as if they belong to others. Therefore, we blame other people for what we don't want to feel and we judge and condemn them. Through this process, there is often aggression, attack and violence that we feel justified to exert.

In some form or another, the mind has given us the illusion that we can escape from suffering. These methods of avoidance never give the results expected. Sooner or later we will eventually feel the pain that we are trying to avoid either physically or emotionally or both. Freedom from pain is found in the exact opposite of resisting it. *In surrendering, you will find peace.*

Allowing

Throughout this guidebook, specific tools are given to alleviate the resistance that may arise when recalling your life story. I have used these tools myself and found them to be very helpful and even necessary for my own healing. The process of *allowing* has been used by many teachers in multiple forms. I share with you the one method that gave me the best results. The mind will resist the simplicity of it and will call it *stupid*. Just know that it works!

Sit quietly, alone, and allow sufficient time for this process. By feeling pressured with time, it could be a clever way of avoiding a memory to surface. If possible, play some peaceful music in the background. Breathe deeply and simply allow your body to feel any feeling and/or sensation that it may experience each time you search your memory. If you are having some discomfort in your body, know that it is perfectly normal. Say the following affirmation:

Allowing

I allow myself to remember

After saying the affirmation, notice how your body feels. If you are feeling comfortable and you are allowing memories to surface, continue on, to the next step of "remembering." If you are feeling uncomfortable and resisting the process of allowing, realize that it is not necessary for you to understand the reasons why you are resisting, just allow the resistance to occur and do the following:

Answer yes or no to the following three questions without analyzing them. Keep repeating the same process until you feel free of the resistance in your body.

1. Could I welcome the feeling of resistance as best I can in this moment? Yes or no?
If yes, go to #2. If no, go to #1A.

1A. Ask yourself: "Would I rather keep this feeling of resistance or would I rather be free?" Remember that what you resist is what creates the pain. Are you willing to let it go? In other words: Am I willing to let go of the resistance? Then make sure to answer "yes". The next question to ask yourself is when can I let it go? Simply reply, *now*. Then breathe and just let go. Notice if your body feels somewhat lighter and freer from the resistance. Repeat this process a few more times until you feel the resistance dissolving. When you feel confident to move forward, go to the "Remembering" process.

2. Could I allow myself to let it go? Yes or no?
If yes, go to #3. If no, go to 1A.

3. When Could I let go of the resistance? Simply answer, *now*.

This process really works, I have done it dozens of times for many situations in my life. Allowing versus resisting will set you free. *What we resist, persist*. Refer back to the allowing process each time you find yourself resisting any other steps in the guidebook.

Remembering

Place a photo of yourself or you with your family and say the following:

Remembering
I vividly remember my childhood

This affirmation may stir up some emotions in you, such as fear. Acknowledge the emotion that you are feeling and if necessary, review the process of "Allowing".

When you are ready, sit quietly, close your eyes and allow the first memory of your childhood to come to mind and answer the following six questions:

1. What do you see?
2. How old are you?
3. Who is there with you?
4. How do you feel?
5. What is happening?
6. Where do you feel discomfort in your body if any?

Take a moment to write down as many details as you can remember. If you only see colors versus events or people, write that as well. It is valuable information. If you don't have any visual memory but you are experiencing sensations in your body, write those sensations to questions 4, 5 and 6.

When I recalled my first memory, my stomach and upper abdomen areas were reacting very strongly to my internal turmoil. I was feeling actual pain in both areas of my body. In the past, I avoided those sensations but I found that, by no longer resisting the pain, I was able to move forward. So, I strongly urge you to feel through the experience and allow it. Of course if you undergo excruciating emotional or physical pain, stop and please get help. But if you are feeling confident in moving forward, I can assure you that eventually, the discomfort will dissolve.

In answering question 6, write the areas in your body where you are feeling uneasiness. Even a slight sensation is worth noting.

In Appendix A, at the end of the workbook, there is a list of feelings that may help you recognize what you are sensing. Please take a moment to familiarize yourself with it.

In part 1 of my book, my first memory was of when I was 2 years old, I encourage you to remember as far back as you can between the age of 0 to 7 years old.

Inviting The Subconscious Mind

Once I recollected some events from my childhood, more memories resurfaced for me. The same might happen to you. Write below the subsequent memories that are coming up. Trust that your subconscious mind is bringing these memories for healing. Review the process of allowing if necessary.

Repeat the following affirmation:

Inviting

I am inviting my subconscious mind to reveal the memories that are beneficial for my remembrance

Now, go back again in time to where you were living as a child and continue to describe your experience:
1. What do you see?
2. How old are you?
3. Who is there with you?
4. How do you feel?
5. What is happening?
6. Where do you feel discomfort in your body if any?

Let's repeat this process until you are about 7 years old. Write the memories as they come to you if you don't remember your age it does not matter just write your experiences as they unfold in your mind while trying to go back in time as far as you can.

Honoring Your Inner Child

I am comforting my inner child
I am trusting my inner child
I am healing my inner child

While I was reliving my childhood's memories, I was feeling very unsafe, insecure, and afraid. I realized that my inner child was suffering. She needed to trust me in order to reveal her most intimate feelings to me. It became impossible for me to continue the writing of my book. To move forward, I had to acknowledge her. As I was looking at a picture of her, I promised her that I was going to take care of her, no matter what. I reassured her that she was now free to speak and that her feelings were of great importance to me. I held her close to my heart and comforted her. Every night before I went to sleep, I looked at her picture and asked her to visit me in my dreams and let me know how I could help her.

One night, I had such a dream. I, the adult was holding my little girl's hand and we were both running into a field of grass and flowers. We were both laughing and felt so carefree. When I woke up with that vision in mind, I understood its profound message. She was finally trusting me and together we were running towards freedom. No more sufferings…only laughter. I felt compelled to write her a letter which I am including here:

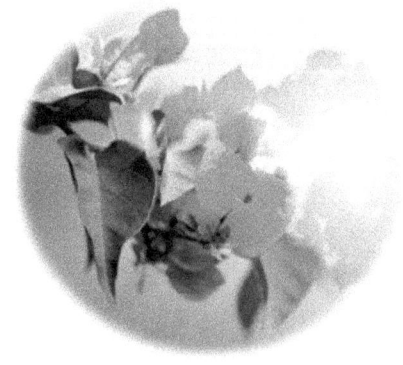

My little girl:

I dreamed about you last night and for the first time I heard your laughter. I was holding your hand and we were both running into the fields. There was a blue sky above us, and the sun felt warm like a summer day. There was even a breeze in the air. I just woke up and the sound of your voice is still fresh in my mind. Thank you for visiting me this way. I feel so honored that you are trusting me, as I know how difficult this is for you. I promise you that I will never let you down and I will always be as courageous as you are! If I make a mistake along the way, just let me know how you feel and I will correct it immediately. I never want you to suffer again and I will do all that I can to make you feel safe with me. Your birthday is coming up in a few months. What do you want? Can you tell me? Please make a list and share it with me. I will give you every little thing your heart desires as you deserve the very best. In the meantime, I am preparing a surprise for you. I'm giving you a little hint: it has something to do with you…your life story is being written. The surprise is yet to come, we shall see when I present it to you. I never met anyone like you! You are in fact the most amazing person in the whole world and I love you so much!

Thank you for letting me honor you.

Letter to your inner child

It is very important that you write your own letter to your inner child. May be you will even feel inspired to record with your own voice what you would say to that inner child that wants to be comforted by you.

Speak of all the qualities you see in him/her. Congratulate your inner child in the healing steps he/she is taking.

Once the inner child knows that he/she will be protected by you, he/she will continue to reveal things to you in the most beautiful way. Finally he/she is being recognized, loved, respected and accepted. That little child will become your best ally in your healing journey.

Speak to your inner child daily during your healing process. Ask him/her what is needed from you. Reassure your inner child that he/she is safe with you, that you are the parent now and you will never hurt him/her. Soon, you will greatly benefit from the healing potential of this daily interaction with your inner child.

Take your inner child with you and play. This is especially important if you didn't play enough as a child.

I encourage you to continue this process with your inner child each time you are feeling intense emotions surfacing for healing. It is a balm for your wounds. Cherish those moments.

One day, my inner child spoke to me again through a dream and said: Now, I have another plan for you. Remember the dream that you had? It is time now, hold my hand and I will guide you through this journey. I am wiser than you are as I still have the innocence of a child and the wisdom of the soul that lives within me. It is your time to trust me now. Can you continue this journey with me? "Absolutely," I replied without hesitation. When I woke up, I wrote the dream down and I took myself out on a date to breakfast. I then drove to the closest flower shop and bought the most beautiful bouquet of flowers that I could find. When I came back home, I put the flowers in an elegant vase and put them in front of a picture of myself when I was 3 years old, that was displayed on my nightstand. I kneeled in front of that little girl's picture and joining my hands as in prayer, I said to her, "My little girl, from this day on, I will honor you. I will honor your words when you speak to me. I will respect your pain when you poke at me as a reminder to take care of you. I will write your story as if it was the most beautiful story I had ever heard and I will tell it to everyone that wants to hear it and know about you. I will remember that you like to play and laugh with friends. I promise you, that I will forgive myself if I make mistakes along the way and won't beat myself down anymore. I will look at you in the deep of your blue eyes and seek the wisdom your soul is teaching me. And every night when I go to sleep, I will say good night and ask you to guide me in the realm of angels where you live and where you can teach me the path of love and compassion for myself and for others that served a purpose in my life. I will thank them for my healing tears and see the beauty in them as I continue to discover my own. Show me the way. I am ready."

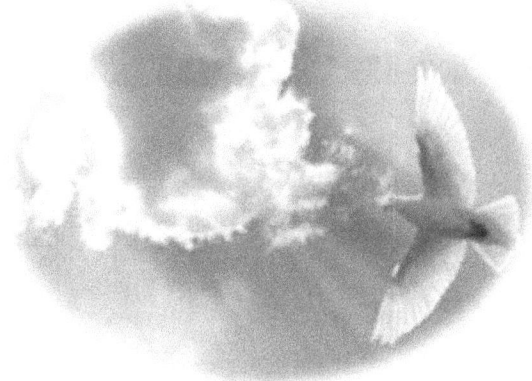

A dove just came by my window and flew away as I finished writing these words. Maybe I am free to fly now...

Honoring Your Emotions

I am honoring all my emotions and as I release them,
healing is occurring within me

Allow yourself to feel the emotions once denied to you.

If you were raised in an abusive home mourn the childhood you never had.

If you were not allowed to feel anger, that anger needs to be released now in a constructive way toward the abuser and not yourself through guilt.

List here the reasons why you are angry and with whom:
I am angry at:
Because of:
List what you want from them:

Share your feelings with someone you trust; a therapist, a friend or simply write a letter or letters to the people that caused you pain even if they are no longer alive. Do a ceremonial and burn the letters as you visualize releasing all your emotions into smoke.

Interact with the persons on an imaginary level and share with them what you couldn't say.

If necessary, to express anger, use physical movements such as screaming, kicking a chair, hitting a pillow. I recommend holding back the tears. Use crying for the pain and sadness that you feel, but not to express anger.

Underneath anger there is hurt and fear. Feel all the layers.

Ask yourself throughout the day: How am I feeling? What is that emotion that I feel? Why am I having this emotion? Write in your journal. Comfort yourself and your inner child.

Don't judge your thoughts, just be conscious of them.

List what behaviors you are no longer willing to tolerate.

Decide what needs to be done.

Make a list of the qualities you admire and decide to be around people that have those qualities.

Don't ask why. You immediately become a victim. Why do I keep repeating the same patterns? What's wrong with me? I can't believe I did this again?

Notice your internal dialogue and change it immediately. It takes 21 days to reframe a pathway into the brain. When you notice that your internal dialogue is negative, get up and do something...anything to make you get out of the victimization role and self-sabotage talk.

Praise yourself daily.

If you were an abused child, recognize that the tendency to get involved in abusive relationships is not your fault. Give as much understanding to yourself as you give others.

You can use a technique called EFT (Emotional Freedom Technique) to help you release emotions and create new empowering ones. Reiki energy healing is very beneficial in activating the natural healing process of the physical, emotional and spiritual aspects of oneself.

Guilt, (especially neurotic guilt) is when you feel guilty, rather than accepting the fact that you were helpless as a child. When you take on the guilt or shame of the person who victimized you, you may use some form of therapy to release that anger, otherwise it will continue to be turned inward and somehow, you will continue to punish yourself.

It is natural as a child, when you experience loss or trauma, to respond with fear or hurt. If you lived in an environment where feelings were not allowed to be expressed, you eventually feel as if you caused the loss or trauma and consequently feel shame and guilt. When fear or hurt can't be expressed, you may become angry. If expressing anger was unacceptable by your parents, you probably became very confused, sad, shamed, and empty. You may have turned that anger inward towards yourself or you may have an explosive temper as an adult. It is also possible that you have blocked all the feelings you were not allowed to feel and became numb.

As you become an adult, you are faced with options to either hold everything in until it becomes unbearable and become physically or emotionally sick, or numb the pain with alcohol, drugs, food, or some other form of addiction. Since none of those options will serve your best interest, facing and feeling what you were not allowed to feel as a child is the safest path toward recovery.

Choosing the Heroic path

Choosing

I am choosing to live the heroic path and live an inspiring life

Today, you are free to make a choice to either follow the path of the victim/martyr or take the heroic path which will lead you ultimately to freedom. Which one do you choose?

The path of the Victim/Martyr leads to:

Hurt -→ Anger -→Resentment and/or Guilt-→Unawareness leads to -→Chronic illness -→Pain and suffering inflicted to oneself and others.

The path of the Hero/Heroine leads to:

Hurt --→ Anger -→Awareness leads to -→Commitment to heal -→Experiencing and telling your story -→Completing -→Resolution, Integration -→Growth, healing -→Contentment -→Joy, love, peace.

Honoring Your Body

I honor my body
I trust the wisdom of my body
I understand my beautiful body

There is no greater agony then bearing an untold story inside of you" Maya Angelou.

You bear your untold story in your body. Your inner child remembers how your body felt. As an adult, it is crucial to allow the stored emotions to be recognized in your body.

I recalled the physical symptoms I experienced as a child created by the emotion of fear: Nose bleeds, depression, strep throats with fever of 104 degrees, constipation, anxiety, internal bleeding, cysts, tumor, hemorrhoids, anemia, diarrhea, and later in life heart problems.

Fear experienced to such an extreme degree (such as in the case of my sister Yvanne) often leads to self-destructive behaviors. At a very young age, Yvanne became addicted to alcohol, later to prescription drugs and finally ended her own life at the age of 52, after 3 unsuccessful previous suicide attempts. She also had various allergies, asthma, suffered from migraine headaches, depression, and anxiety. Both my sister and I, in our early thirties, had a total hysterectomy.

My oldest sister was affected by depression, anxiety, breast cancer, migraines, addiction to pain killer due to the migraines. She is a 3rd stage breast cancer survivor.

List here any past or current physical symptoms including surgeries:
Age:
Condition:

On the left side of the following illustration, write down all of the emotions that you experienced.

On the right side, write down all the physical symptoms corresponding to the area of the body where you experienced pain or illness.

Your body has its own inner intelligence; allow it to speak to you.
You will refer to this chart again and see the correlation between your body, your emotions and the chakra system explained in the next pages.

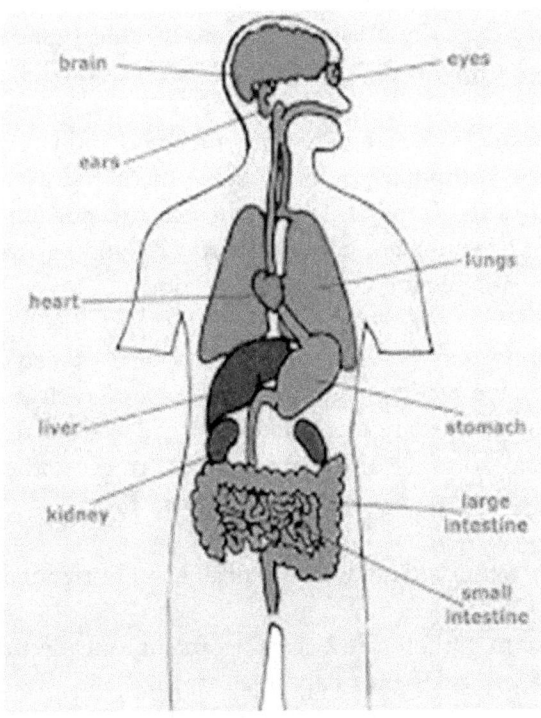

Harmonizing Body and Mind

My body and mind are in perfect harmony

Spiritual Centers

So far, we have concentrated on your physical and emotional states; however, you are also a spiritual being, having a human experience. In the process of healing, the four aspects of body, mind, soul and spirit are addressed:

I recognize that I am body, mind soul and spirit
I allow Divine Guidance into my life

Meaning of the Chakras: The word chakra comes from Sanskrit and means wheel or disk of energy. The spinning of those wheels of energy is created by the presence of consciousness (spirit) within the physical body.

The chakra system is a gate between your mind and your body. Think of yourself as a computer, the body being the hardware and the mind being the software (programs). As the electric current allows your computer to communicate between hardware and software, so is the energy system connecting your mind and body.

For the purpose of this guidebook, although we have more than seven chakras, we will concentrate only on the seven *main* wheels of energy. The 7 chakras are identified from the bottom up as the root, spleen or sacral, solar plexus, heart, throat, 3 rd eye and crown on top of the head. (*Please refer to the chart on Appendix B*)

Your chakras gather energy both vertically and horizontally.

A chakra system gathers the energy from the outside processes it in the inside of the body and expresses it out again. Referring to the computer language, the energy from the outside is the information you are receiving from those around you (input). You process that input inside your body (the processor) and you express it into your physical world (output). A long time ago when I was a programmer/analyst we used the expression: garbage in, garbage out. That is so true!

Now, let's look at how the chakra system gathers the energy vertically. There are 2 currents of energy flow:

Upward: From the earth rising upward, step by step through each of the seven chakra to the liberation process, enlightenment.

Downward: Consciousness descending towards the earth into the manifestation process.

Moving with the upward current, increased freedom may be gained from the limitations of the physical world, new possibilities arise and it is the path of freedom from the physical form.

Moving downward is the flow of manifestation. You may have an idea about a project but it won't take form until you bring it down to the physical plane. It is the path of enjoyment in the physical form.

How your emotions affects your body

On the previous pages, you recorded your emotions and the physical illnesses or conditions that were a consequence of your emotional state of being. Now, let's look further into how emotions affect not only your body, but your chakra system as well.

Emotions are composed of feelings and sensations that you feel in your body. They are a powerful source of information about the general state of well-being.

Following is a brief description of each of the main chakras listing issues or areas of concern when a specific chakra is out of balance... that is, when the energy flow is blocked. Over time it may cause diseases in the body. Use the following information provided to assess your overall state of being both physically, emotionally and spiritually. Look at the characteristics of each of the chakras and make note of the ones that applies to you. It is possible that each chakra is affected. By addressing your emotions and taking the necessary measures to heal them, it is possible to reverse the physical imbalances in the body and restore the flow of energy.

In the Chinese system, everything ultimately boils down to energy, a view which modern Western physics is beginning to verify. Therefore, the Chinese approach to human health and physiology accounts not only for the effects of obvious visible substances such as microbes and toxins, blood and bile, but also for the invisible and even more pervasive influences of emotions and energies that have a direct impact on the human energy.

You may circle all the conditions applying to you and see which chakra needs balancing.

Chakra 1: Root

The Root Chakra is red, and located at the tailbone. It is masculine in nature, and associated with the adrenal glands.

Primary characteristics include survival, security, stability, and the ability to meet one's basic needs.

Possible emotions/feelings: Fear, worry, anxiety, depression, frustration and anger.

Physical areas of the body affected when this chakra is out of balance:

Colon, knees, kidneys, legs, feet, bones

Possible physical symptoms: Constipation or diarrhea, nervous diseases, neck pain, arthritis

Chakra 2: Spleen or Sacral

The Sacral Chakra is orange, and located just below the navel. It is feminine in nature, and associated with the reproduction glands.

Primary characteristics include sexuality, creativity, reproduction, emotionality, and adaptability.

Possible emotions/feelings: Guilt is the primary cause of dysfunction in this chakra. Jealousy, cruelty, loneliness, inadequacy, helplessness, hopelessness, worries, numbness, restlessness, laziness, excessive mood swings, angry easily.

Physical areas of the body affected when this chakra is out of balance:

Ovaries, testicules and genitals, womb, lower back, hips, pelvis, colon, bladder, small intestines, kidneys, skin.

Possible physical imbalances: Cancer of the colon, bladder infections, ovarian cysts, low sexual desire or sexual addictions, bowel problems, impotence, back pain, weight problems, reproductive issues.

Chakra Three: Solar Plexus

The Solar Plexus is yellow, and located below the breast bone. It is masculine in nature, and associated with the pancreas.

Primary characteristics include personal power, confidence, and mental agility.

Possible emotions/feelings: Shame is the primary emotion causing imbalance in this chakra. Fear, anxiety, low self-esteem, lack will power and self-confidence, guilt, communication difficulties, feels like a failure, depression, mood swings, laziness, cruelty, not willing to trust intuition.

Physical areas of the body affected when this chakra is out of balance:

Stomach, liver, gall bladder, intestines.

Possible physical symptoms: Hyperactive or lack of energy, poor digestion, mental fatigue, weight problems.

Chakra Four: Heart

The Heart Chakra is green, and located at the heart. It has feminine qualities, and is associated with the thymus gland.

Primary characteristics include loving yourself and others, compassion, kindness, and a sense of peace.

Possible emotions/feelings: Grief is the main emotion causing imbalance in this chakra. Jealousy, possessiveness, insecurity, selfishness, demanding, fears commitments, grief, loneliness, being a martyr, being a pleaser, poor boundaries, codependency, critical, intolerant, isolation, lack of empathy, fear of intimacy.

Physical areas of the body affected when this chakra is out of balance:

Heart, lungs, circulatory system, shoulders, arms, ribs/breasts, upper back, chest, blood, immune system.

Possible physical symptoms: Respiratory problems, asthma, high blood pressure, heart problems.

Chakra Five: Throat

The Throat Chakra is blue, and is located in the throat center. The throat chakra carries masculine qualities and is associated with the thyroid.

Primary characteristics include standing and speaking your truths, expressing oneself creatively, and maintaining integrity in all areas of living.

Possible emotions/feelings: Depression, loneliness, emotional unrest, lack of satisfaction, gossip, lack creativity, difficulties in self-expression, easily angry, arrogant, talks too much with very little substance or fear of speaking, needs to be in control, very stubborn, excessive shyness, stuttering, speaking with a small voice or high voice.

Physical areas of the body affected when this chakra is out of balance:

Thyroid, neck, shoulder, mouth, jaw, throat, gums, cervical spine, esophagus, teeth, ears.

Possible physical symptoms: Muscle tension, inflammations, colds, visual and auditory problems, depression, loneliness, hypochondria, hypertension, neck tension, low energy, sore throat, swollen glands, tight jaws, TMJ, speech problems, teeth and gums problems, stiffness in neck and shoulders.

Chakra Six: Third eye

The Third Eye or Brow Chakra is indigo in color, and located above the brow, between the eyes. Feminine in nature, and associated with the pineal gland.

Primary characteristics of the brow chakra include wisdom, imagination, vision, perception, and intuition. (*Imagination is more important than knowledge. Albert Einstein*)

Possible emotions/feelings: Closed thinking, learning disabilities, resistance to new and/or different ideas, lack focus, identify with the drama of your life, obsessive thinking, feeling disconnected from other people, lack of imagination, insensitivity, excessive skepticism, denial, obsessions.

Physical areas of the body affected when this chakra is out of balance:

Memory, vision, hearing, sinuses, migraines, sleep disturbances.

Possible physical symptoms: Exhaustion, sleep problems, headaches, eye and sinus problems, nervous behaviors, paranoia, neurological disturbances including, multiple sclerosis, Parkinson's disease, polio, brain tumor, strokes, learning disabilities, nightmares, hallucinations. Extreme sensitivity to light and sound.

Chakra Seven: Crown

The Crown Chakra is violet or white, located just above the crown of the head, and is associated with the pituitary gland. Since this is not a "bodily" chakra, it is unified, rather than associated with feminine or masculine aspects.

The primary characteristic of the crown chakra is connection to the divine or universal life force for spiritual development.

(He who knows others is wise, but he who knows himself is enlightened. Lao Tzu)

Possible emotions/feelings: Depression, closed to all spirituality, lack accountability, lack of self-awareness, confusion, disconnection from spirit, excessive attachments, spiritual cynicism, a closed mind, rigid belief systems, need to be perfect, make lots of judgments, righteous.

Physical areas of the body affected when this chakra is out of balance:

Pituitary gland at the base of the brain affecting the nervous system and the endocrine system.

Possible physical symptoms: Tumors, kidneys and bladder infections, concussion, nervous system, depression.

Now, that you identified your emotions, your physical symptoms, the chakra or chakras in need of your attention, where do you go from here?

Blindly, throughout my life, with different people and different situations, I kept repeating the same patterns causing me to suffer. Subconsciously, without awareness in my mind, I had created a pathway to react to fear (in its many forms) since I was 2 years old and did not have a way out.

In June of 2010, I almost died. I had a condition called supraventricular tachycardia. SVTs by definition are caused by abnormal circuitry in the heart that creates a loop of overlapping signals. In my case, the signal to the heart was caught in a loop and couldn't find its way out. That condition reflected back to me how I was living my life at that time.

I was walking in a labyrinth swirling and unable to find a way out.

I had to reprogram my mind to come to my rescue. My old program was putting my body under a tremendous amount of stress, feeling and reacting as if I was under attack and in need of defending myself. Of course this belief was reinforced by the world around me.

My willingness to heal myself led me to the work of a few teachers: one of them being Dr. David H. Hawkins who published the world acclaimed book Powervs. Force. It was fascinating to learn about the different levels of consciousness which, I included in this guidebook. Refer to appendix C.

What is the connection between Body, Mind, and Spirit? What follows is a recapitulation of notes that I took from different sources and from different teachers such as Dr. Hawkins' work on consciousness and Eckhart Tolle's work on the ego. It is important to note that I only give you my understanding of such complex subjects. I highly recommend that you read the work of those authors yourself. In the interim, it is my hope that you may find it helpful to get an overview on those subjects.

A body can't experience itself without the mind. (A body is experienced by the mind via the brain).

The mind is the human consciousness that originates in the brain and is manifested especially in thought, perception, emotion, will, memory and imagination.

As a result, it is important to understand that the mind is a highly intricate network of different mental events and emotional conditions. It is a highly advanced and sophisticated computer that no one has as of yet, been able to duplicate and fully understand.

So, our thoughts are part of the human mind. These thoughts are mainly unconscious. Unconscious thoughts are like a program running in your mind (the computer). When you say *I think*, you are actually hearing a voice inside your head speaking to you. So, a thought happens to you just like when you say *I am walking*, you are in fact being walked by your mind telling you to move one leg in front of the other.

The mind can't experience itself without consciousness. What is consciousness?

It is conscious, eternal, immortal, timeless and unmanifested. It is the intelligence that creates forms (our bodies) into a manifested universe (our planet) in order to experience itself. All of us are part of the consciousness, spirit, or God if you prefer. A soul is an individuality of consciousness choosing to experience and learn in order to evolve through an earthly experience as in the case of humans on this planet. When consciousness enters the form (the body through the mind) it loses itself into the form and thinks it is separate from its Creator. So, consciousness becomes unconscious of itself. Therefore, human beings are unconscious about being consciousness itself.

This separation is what is called the *ego*. The ego then, thinks of itself as a separate entity and becomes completely identified with the mind with the aspect of thinking. Thinking is only one small aspect of the totality of consciousness. When the ego is in place, we suffer depending on our level of identification with the egoic mind.

When you experience joy, peace, love, you are then experiencing another aspect of consciousness.

It may help if you see the mind split in two: one side of the mind being the ego which is to live in a world of form and illusions, fear and guilt. The other side of the mind is Spirit which is living in a world of Truth, love, peace and joy.

Emotions are the body's reactions to what you hold in mind, your programming and your thoughts. Emotions can also be triggered by an event. Depending on how that event is translated and interpreted in your mind as good or bad, your body will then react accordingly. Remember the body experiences itself through the mind. It is in fact possible to experience in your body the same emotion you felt 10 years ago by simply *thinking* about it as if it was happening right now.

The purpose of your life is to become conscious, which means to be aware, to be awake, to know that you are consciousness into form and that you can create a reality according to your level of consciousness. You can create unconsciously with the ego or you can create consciously by being aware of your thoughts that will dictate your actions. Masters such as Paramahansa Yogananda have told us that a thought is even more important than action because it is the force that instigates the action. So, a thought ignited with the emotion (fear, anger, love, compassion etc.) creates fire and you choose how to use the flame. It can serve or destroy. Thought + emotion = Action.

The ego was created for survival in this dimension and now that the old is being dissolved for our awakening, the more dysfunctional the ego may become in the same way that a caterpillar becomes dysfunctional just before it transforms into a butterfly. The ego, by its idea of separateness, reinforces the belief in separation and therefore competes with others, love to argue about who is right and who is wrong, who is better or less than and often creates pain and suffering. Great spiritual teachers have told us that there is a new consciousness coming to earth, and now more than ever before, humanity has an incredible opportunity to become aware of one's divinity, having a physical experience. By this awareness, one can create consciously what one chooses to manifest.

It is also important to realize that the mind is also subject to the collective consciousness. Think of the collective consciousness as the collection of minds (computers) hooked to a giant database where all information is available to access and where all the individual minds, thinking at the same level, are being reinforced by the power of the collective. When your individual beliefs match the collective, you are being transported into a very powerful energy field that will make your desired reality happen.

Wars are created in that energy field as well as peace. What do you want to create?

Consequently, it is very important to recognize your level of consciousness to help you achieve the reality you desire in your life. As you raise your level of consciousness, you will be aligned with the field of the collective as well. If you align yourself with anger, you will reinforce the anger in you. If you align yourself with the field of love, you will increase the field of love within yourself.

Your beliefs become your reality. You will make decisions, and take actions based on your beliefs. If I believe I have an enemy, I may attack to defend myself. If I believe I don't have enemies, the need to attack or defend dissolve. There will be peace on earth. That is *not* the way of the ego, as the ego strives on opposition.

One can't create consciousness through unconsciousness so how does one become conscious?

You achieve consciousness by becoming aware of your thoughts, your programming and the power of your thinking in relationship to the emotions that they produce. By being aware of your individual level of consciousness, you can now make better choices.

While writing my life story, I was vacillating at different levels of consciousness since I was not completely done with the letting go process. Unconsciously, *I still had layers* of resentment in my heart about my father and I was blaming him for my sister's choice to end her life. I had to find a way to reconcile these emotions in my mind, body and soul. I eventually reached a level of understanding and acceptance that transcended to a level of reason and wisdom which calibrates at 400. Please refer to Appendix C.

For the sake of clarity, let me say that I am totally against abuse in all its forms, but without having a different kaleidoscope view, one may be unable to move forward and get stuck in the blaming game. My mind (the ego) was giving me all the justifications to remain angry, resentful and unforgiving. That is not the path I desired to walk on. Therefore, to move forward in my healing journey, I had to be open to a different perspective in my life story to ultimately view my soul's perspective. You can only fix a problem at the *level **above** the one it was created.*

As difficult as it may be, allow yourself to move away from the judgments that will come up in your mind.

It takes a lot of courage to step away from blaming others that have wronged you. If you want to get unstuck from that energy, allow yourself to perceive your story in different angles which is offer to you here:

Willingness

I am willing to perceive my story differently

Healing is found in the desire to change our perception or opinion about a situation or a person.

In order to have a different perspective about the characters in your life story, I suggest the following:

First, be open and receptive to the idea that however wrong was done to you by those people, they did all that they could have done at the time. At least recognize that you may not have all the information needed about their lives that could help you understand them better.

Remember each time you close a door; you close a door to yourself.

As an example for you to follow, this is the process that helped me to shift my perspective. In your process, replace "father" or "mother" with the character(s) that wronged you. Complete the perspective process in your journal. But first, you must identify your goals, recall how you felt and identify the characters in your story.

My goals were the following: Forgive my parents and empower myself through feelings of joy, peace, self-love and respect.

How did I feel? Abused, abandoned, unloved, neglected, unprotected.

Characters in my story: Father, mother.

What was the problem: Abuse

Father:

What are his problems? Alcoholism, inferiority complex, shyness, lack of education, possible abuse by his own father, money issues, stress.

What did he want to achieve? Discipline

How did he achieve that? Through the use of physical and emotional abuse.

Do you know why he chose those methods? ignorance, cruelty, it gave him a sense of power and control, he was part of the collective consciousness belief that abusing your children meant to discipline them. He had resentment about having daughters instead of boys.

Circumstances at the time: Money issues, alcohol usage and stress.

Do you think, knowing his situation, that he did all he could have done? My father was removed from school by his father when he was around 11 years old to work on a farm every day. Although he had a brilliant mind, he was not given the opportunity to further his education. He once told us that his father beat him up with the belt when he 19 years old because he was late coming home. I am assuming that there was resentment in his heart against his father.

Can you try to understand the motive for his behavior? I believe that my father was in love with my mother, but did not want the responsibility of having children. He reverted to drinking to repress the anger and resentment that he never dealt with. Assuming that he didn't want children, he was forced to fill out those unwanted obligations. That was the price to pay to be with my mother since having children was part of marriage. My father wanted a son and resented having 3 daughters. He possibly hated himself so much, that his only escape was to inflict the same level of pain to another as he was feeling inside. He projected on us, his view of himself. I often thought about how painful it must have been to be my father.

Can you forgive him? I choose to forgive him so that I can be happy and free.

Forgiveness is a choice. You may choose forgiveness and freedom or revenge and hell. Which do you choose?

Mother:

What are her problems? Depression, stress, martyrdom, enabler, money issues.

What did she want to achieve? Discipline

How did she achieve that? By encouraging the discipline measures

Do you know why she chose those methods? She was part of the same consciousness beliefs on discipline. She was depressed and helpless. She may have not wanted children, but her religious beliefs didn't allow her to use birth control. Since I know that my conception was an accident, I am assuming that my sister, Yvanne was also.

Circumstances at the time: Money issues, stress, depression.

Do you think, knowing her situation, that she did all she could have done? Yes. Considering her depressed state and the helplessness she felt. She didn't want 3 children and she probably was resentful as well. My father's drinking problem and irresponsibleness added to her sense of helplessness. I don't know much about her parents except that her mother was a very cold and unaffectionate person. My mother delegated the discipline to her husband, like most parents did at the time. Being unable to protect herself from her own state of victimization, she permitted her husband to victimize her children. We felt like she did, unprotected and victimized.

Can you forgive her? Yes, because my own state of mind is to release myself from victim hood. I choose happiness and empowerment.

In your current life situation, answer the following:

How do you think the character feels today?

Has the character tried to reconcile with you? If so, what was the outcome?

What is your relationship with that character today?

What do you want for yourself? Make sure you don't try to have the character do something for you. Choose what you want. An example of choosing what you want would be to write a letter, call or meet in order to express what you feel without accusations.

What is your life today? Which role are you playing in your current life? Are you a victim? Are you an abuser? Are you an enabler?

What are the problems in your current life?

With who?

How do you feel?

Is this problem similar to the one you lived in your childhood?

Describe the similarity?

Write down the positive qualities of your father and circle the ones you have in common with him.

Write down the negative traits of you father and circle the ones you have in common with him.

Write down the positive traits of your partner and circle the ones similar to your father or mother.

Write down the negative traits of your partner and circle the ones familiar with both of your parents.

Do you recognize the similarity between all the characters in your story?

Now, take a look at your life can you see where the similarities intertwine?

As an example, like my mother, I became a victim. But, what blew me away was the recognition that I was unconsciously choosing my partners *to heal the relationship that I had with my father.*

I had to come to the sickening realization that not only was I not going to get my needs met from my partner but that my partner was destined to wound me in the very same way I was wounded in my childhood. It is a very painful discovery. The exciting part comes in when you realize the reason why you chose that partner which is seeking to heal the hidden part of you, the part of you that you are trying to ignore, the childhood wounds. The main reason why people move from relationships to relationships is because it becomes too painful to deal with those hidden issues. So, we blame our partner and we move on to the next.

I need to add that most importantly I needed to learn to forgive myself for my so-call mistakes. I built resentment against myself because of the choices that I made and I didn't realize that I needed to forgive myself for them. Once, I clearly understood that I was seeking to heal those unhealed parts of me, it made perfect sense and I was able to move forward in my healing. It is important to recognize that a girl's father or a boy's mother image provides her or him with an unconscious model for all future romantic encounters. Your partner mirrors back to you, your wounded child.

Your Sacred Soul Journey

Your soul entered your body to come into this dimension to experience, learn, grow and manifest the aspect of your divinity. Your soul will leave your body at a pre-determined time when your mission is accomplished. You will continue to exist in another dimension, or you may choose to come back here on earth and reincarnate in a new body to have a complete different experience according to what you choose to learn next time. If the concept of reincarnation is new to you, it may be beneficial for you to get informed on the subject. Plenty of research and evidence have been confirmed on the subject.

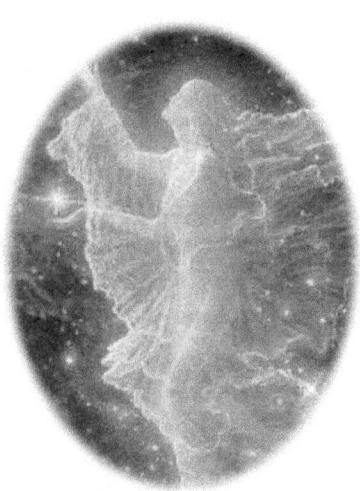

My purpose is not to convince you about reincarnation or that you have a soul, but it may help you to have a different perspective in your life when you realize that you chose your own family and circumstances. By adding your soul's view, you may gain a deeper understanding of your life's lessons.

At some point in our lives, it helps to recognize that we are a soul having a human experience. We study the body and the mind but so often we ignore the soul, when in fact the three aspects need to be addressed for a full recovery and understanding of our lives. We also need to "own up" to the fact that on a soul level, we signed up for this assignment.

My soul's view is the following:

Although I don't remember my past lives,(by the way most people don't as it would defeat the purpose of learning what we came here to experience) I believe that I chose to experience fear in order to experience its opposite, love. Self love, that is. In some cases, and not in all cases, the soul evolution process is often experienced or learned through an opposite force. In my case, if my soul chose to overcome fear would it make sense to be born into a family where I could experience that? From this understanding, it became much easier to move up the scale towards acceptance and wisdom, which lead me to the path of love.

Forgiveness came naturally in the understanding that there was nothing to forgive, since I could no longer accuse. How could I accuse and condemn my father since I had chosen him. I was also blaming him for my sister's death. How could I? She had also chosen him as her father.

What follows is a brief description of the levels of consciousness. By understanding each level, it will help you tremendously in your self-growth process. I compiled information that you can easily follow below, but for a greater understanding I highly recommend that you read Power-vs-Force by Dr. Hawkins.

Mapping your level of Consciousness

The levels of consciousness vary between 20, the lowest level, up to 1,000 which is the level of enlightenment. You may refer to appendix C.

I will provide a description of each level, starting with the lowest level.

Keep in mind that the higher the level of consciousness, the less you are subject to react in a stressful way.

Level of shame (1-20): Someone at this level feels **humiliated**, has low self esteem, is paranoid. Common expressions where one vibrates at this level would be when one feels like he/she has "lost face", wishes he/she is invisible, and feels worthless. Some individuals at shame react by becoming overly rigid and/or exhibit neurotic perfectionism. Prolonged periods in the state of shame, leads to elimination (of self and others), such as suicide, turning into serial killers, rapists, moral extremists who apply self righteous judgment onto others. The person's view of life at this state is misery.

Level of guilt (30): Feelings of **blame** and remorse. Used to consciously or subconsciously manipulate into certain forms of thinking and behaviors. Commonly used in our society with public punishment and finger-pointing culture, by religious institutions with preoccupation of "sin" and "salvation". This level cultivates destruction.

Level of apathy (50): A state of **despair** and helplessness. Dependency on others for help. Because this level feels "heavy" and is seen as a burden to others around, many people usually avoid those who are vibrating at these levels. For example, sadly we recognize how the poor and unfortunate have come to be shielded away from the mainstream society. We also frequently see situations where older people are abandoned because they are seen as a liability.

Level of grief (75): Feelings of **regret**, sadness and loss are experienced here. Many people vibrate at this level in times of losses – of loved ones, relationships, possessions, jobs, money, etc. Someone at grief sees discouragement and hopelessness all around the world and in life. Life is a tragedy. Grief is a higher level than apathy, because one starts feeling more energy at this level.

Level of fear (100): Energy at this level is felt as **anxiety**. Common situations of fear would be fear of rejection, fear of failure, fear of uncertainty, fear of challenges, fear of aging, fear of death, fear of loss, fear of strangers. Fear leads to paranoia and can turn into an obsession. At this level, one views everything uncertain as fearful and thus undergoes the state of withdrawal. Thus, fear prevents personal growth from taking place. Someone in the level of fear sees the world as frightening.

Level of desire (125): At the level of desire, the emotion of **craving** becomes dominant. The pursuit of money and status as end goals for a better life dominate this level. Addictions are outputs of desire, such as desire for food, video games, fun, sex, shopping, acquisition of money and power, etc. One becomes looped into enslavement at this level, because desire is never-ending emotion. The life-view is disappointing, which ensues when one cannot obtain what one desires. Desire is a higher level than fear because the desire for something propels people forward to action, rather than withdraw to a corner.

Level of anger (150): The emotion at this level is **hate.** Anger expresses itself as resentment, frustration and even revenge. At the individual level, examples include irritable and volatile behavior, short-temper. The upside of anger is that it has resulted in liberation and great movements in the society; the downside is dangerous behavior and intentional harm that might ensue from it. The process one undergoes is aggression. The life-view here is antagonistic, where one is hostile, unfriendly and acts in opposition/rebellion against others.

Level of pride (175): DR. Hawkins cites **scorn** as the dominant feeling of pride. In our current society, pride is a level that is encouraged and seen as positive – for example, pride of being part of a group, institution, company, nation, religion, race. However, this leads to duality viewpoints, which acts as an invisible force to separate people. For example, nations exist because people identify themselves more with a geographical location rather than a universal identity. Religions exist because people attach themselves to their beliefs of God and values which serve as a separator. On a personal level, people form pride based on possessions and external conditions, and it is vulnerable because such conditions can be removed at any point in time. Pride results in denial and arrogance. At the pride level, one undergoes inflation (of ego) rather than being able to see things objectively.

Level of courage (200): Affirmation is the key emotion here. *This is the separation point between Power and Force,* where one is starts creating change through the use of constructive states of power rather than destructive force. This is the *first waking point* where one starts becoming awaken. At the lower levels before this, the world is seen as hopeless, tragic, frightening, demanding; People from below 200 sees themselves as victims, at the mercy of life and subjected to forces of the external world.

At the courage level, one sees the world as exciting and filled with possibilities. One undergoes *empowerment* here. This marks the start of the active pursuit of growth – where there exists a gap, the person will act to fill it. For example, learning new job skills, embarking on new education, pursuing personal growth. Anything is manageable since the person is able to harness power to deal with situations in life. People in the higher levels greater than 200 recognize that their happiness and life lies within them.

Level of neutrality (250): The emotion at this level is **trust** and safety. Here, people are non-judgmental, objective and able to see things as they truly are. They are not attached to possessions, situations, outcomes and can roll with the punches in life. If they are not able to get something, they are equally happy settling for something else.

This is NOT the same as apathy – the power of neutrality comes from a positive place, where one recognizes his/her inner power and abilities and does not feel the need to prove anything to anyone. The process is one of release (of everything), and the life-view is satisfactory, where anything goes. These people are easy to get along; however they are difficult to engage towards causes and visions because they are detached towards everything.

Level of willingness (310): Optimism runs high here. At Willingness, the individual is open to do anything and everything – he/she is not bound by others' judgments or by limitations. For example, he/she is willing to take on menial jobs if he/she cannot get jobs elsewhere. Someone at Willingness can readily bounce back from set-backs, is easily moldable and genuinely open to everyone. Success follows them easily. The process one undergoes here is of intention (to do anything). At this level you have people who perform extremely well in their careers in corporations, start-ups; however the question then comes as to whether they are investing their energy in the best way.

Level of acceptance (350): Here, one finally realizes that he/she is THE creator and source of his/her life, as opposed to having relegated some part of it to someone else. He/she is (1) aware of the social constructs present in one's life, whether by family, society, nation, religion, work (2) able to discern against (limiting) beliefs, viewpoints and conditioning which he/she is surrounded with and (3) able to consciously craft his/her life above and beyond all these social constructs. Characteristic behavior at this level will be acceptance vs. rejection, seeking for resolutions vs. judging right or wrong, long-term vs. short-term view, engaging on life harmoniously on its terms vs. resisting it, striving for personal excellence and growth. Forgiveness is the dominant emotion. The process one undergoes is transcendence (above what one faces in life). The life-view here is harmonious.

Level of reason (400): The emotion is **understanding** and rationality. One seeks out huge amounts of information and analyzes them to microscopic detail before reaching conclusions. This is where the Noble prize winners, leaders of science and medicine and great thinkers of history calibrate. However, Reason falls into the trap of over intellectualization in concepts and theories. Where differing theories clash and each argument is sound on its own, we reach a blockade, leading to the inability to resolve discrepancies.

Level of love (500): This represents unconditional love – love that is pure, unfaltering, unwavering, not subjected to any external conditions. It is not the same love that is commonly portrayed in mass media, which is rooted in lust, desire, pride, control, addiction, attraction, jealousy and possessiveness. While the media often establishes love and hate as opposite poles, hate is actually rooted from pride (desire for control/possessiveness), and not actual love.

Reverence is the main emotion in the level of (unconditional) love. At this level, duality becomes an illusion; the feeling is one of entirety that rises above separation. Unconditional love is inclusive of everyone and expands beyond self. While reason deals with specific data, love deals with entirety, thus giving rise to the capacity for instantaneous understanding. This aspect is often linked with intuition. The process one undergoes is revelation. The life-view is benign; there is no separation, fear or negativity. Dr. Hawkins claims *only 0.4% of the population (1 in every 250 people) ever reaches this level.*

Level of joy (540): The dominant emotion is **serenity** and compassion. This is the inner joy that arises from every moment of existence rather than from an external source. This is the level where saints, advanced spiritual students and healers dwell. At this level, one is characterized by enormous patience and an unwavering positive attitude in the face of harsh adversities. The world is seen as one of perfection and beauty. Individuals are motivated to dedicate themselves to the benefit of life rather than for specific individuals. Here, the process of transfiguration occurs (emanating of radiance from the person). The life-view the individual holds is completeness (of the world). Near death experiences have the effect of temporarily bumping people into this level.

Level of peace (600): The emotion is **bliss**. At this level, there is no longer any distinction between the observer and the subject. People here become spiritual teachers, great geniuses in their field to effect great contribution for mankind; they typically transcend formal religious structures and replace it with pure spirituality where religions originate from. Perception becomes one of slow motion, suspended in time and space. Everything is perceived as interconnected by an infinite presence. The process one undergoes is illumination. Dr. Hawkins claims *this level is only attained by 1 out of 10 million people.*

Level of enlightenment (700-1000): The emotion is **ineffable**, in other words – inexpressible. This is the pinnacle of the evolution of consciousness of mankind. The greatest people of history have attained this level, such as Krishna, Buddha, Jesus, Mother Theresa.

Here, the body becomes recognized as a tool to project consciousness in. One's existence becomes all encompassing and transcends time and space. The process is described as pure consciousness. The life-view here is simply *is*. In achieving our highest potential and embracing our best lives, we should strive for the highest possible level i.e. enlightenment.

The level of consciousness which you are currently at is a weighted average of the different consciousness levels you operate in.

A person usually vibrates at a default consciousness level and shifts to a couple of levels below and above that level depending on the situation. Every thought, every feeling and every action you have in every situation is rooted from a particular consciousness level; all these can be summed up and averaged to identify the default level you are in. It is rare that someone will maintain an exact same state of consciousness in a given period of time. Even within the same day, you may behave at a certain consciousness in this context and at a totally different consciousness in a different context.

One influence on your consciousness is the stimulus in your life. This includes the situations you are in, the type of people you spend time with, your environment and so on. In times of pressure, one's consciousness level usually gets bumped down a few levels. Depending on how the person recovers from the pressure, his or her default consciousness level might be elevated to a higher level after the encounter.

One can move across different levels of consciousness.

Your consciousness level now does not define what your consciousness will be in the future. It is open to change; it is not static. Each person is open to move across different levels, depending on how he/she (chooses to) evolve in his/her consciousness.

Distinction of levels of Power vs. levels of Force

Dr. Hawkins segmented the consciousness into two main categories – one based in force (<200) and one based in power (>200). People in levels of Force vibrate at a level of fear-based emotions. They are more inclined to exert control over others or themselves (oppression, force, coercion, manipulation, violence) to achieve their desired outcomes. For example, crime, war, governmental passing of certain policies, abuse, or even authoritative leadership/parenting styles. People in levels of Power (love, empathy, and understanding) vibrate at a level of love-based emotions. They are increasingly aligned with the present moment and universe and use that to bring about their desired results.

Each level can be beneficial/detrimental to you, depending on the level you are at.

For example, the state of fear (100) may look quite undesirable if you are at the level of desire (125). However, if you are at the state of guilt (30), being around people at state of fear (100) is actually beneficial for you, as it can help elevate you to a higher level. It is generally more effective when you are around people at higher consciousness levels which are closer to your level (vs. a huge distance ahead), since it is easier for your energy levels to reach resonance with theirs. When the people are too distanced from you in their energies, it may result in detachment and alienation instead.

On the same note, when you elevate yourself to a higher level, it becomes obvious that the lower levels are more limiting. For example, if you are at the level of Pride, you will see how levels of Shame/Guilt/Apathy/Grief/Fear/Desire/Anger bind you down. If you are at the level of Acceptance, you will realize how being at levels of Pride/Courage/Neutrality/Willingness restrain you.

At Courage and Acceptance, one experiences a marked leap in the experience of the world.

An increase in consciousness at any level changes your experience significantly. However, there are two particular levels where one experiences a marked leap vs. the other levels. The first is courage which separates the levels of force (<200) from the levels of power (>200). The second is acceptance, where one recognizes it is he and he himself who is the conscious creator of everything in his life. This is the point where one completely awakens.

What level of consciousness are you at? Which level do you find your thoughts and feelings dominating every day?

Remember that every thought, every belief, every feeling and every action you have is rooted from the level of consciousness you are in. When you shift your level of consciousness, you also change your world views. By staying in touch with the map of consciousness throughout the day, it is possible for you to recognize at any given moment where you are on the map. Strive to move at a higher level is the key.

Surrender

One of the most powerful shifts I felt in my life was when I surrendered to it. One of the definitions of the word surrender is to abandon, to give up the right to something. Before I wrote "Healing the Broken Pieces of My Life", I felt entitled to feel the way that I did. I was entitled to feel the pain, the hurts, the resentment, the anger. Even to some degree, the unforgiveness I held in my heart for all of those that had hurt me. I had the right to all those feelings. It was all justifiable!

After I released the remaining of my negative feelings, I realized that I also felt entitled to peace, joy, love and serenity. All those good feelings that I felt entitled to feel after suffering so much. I became aware of the attachment that I was creating by feeling entitled to happiness. I had to give that up, also.
Why? Because in the event that I would not feel happy, I would create unhappiness, just by wanting it. I had to let go of the right to be happy in order to be happy. So, I did. And, by giving up the attachment to that, I became happier.

In surrendering everything, I reached a level of acceptance and self-love that I never thought was possible. It minimized the chatter in my mind. Did you know that thousand of thoughts, even millions of them are associated with only one single feeling? Depending how long you kept that feeling inside, you have built up over the years a multitude of thoughts surrounding it.

The process of surrendering can be done daily. Try this, tomorrow first thing in the morning say: "Today, I will do my best and I will let go of the outcome." See the miracles coming into your life. Every night before you go to sleep, review any unhealed emotions or new ones you didn't let go of during the day and make a commitment to let them go. By letting go, I mean this:

Allow the feeling to exist. One by one, recognize each feeling that comes up. Don't give it a name, don't condemn it, judge it or resist it. When in touch with a particular feeling, invite more of the same feelings to come up. There is no need to vent about your feelings. This is an internal process.

When you are done with the process of allowing, shift your attention to

something else, don't remain in the negative emotion. Shift your awareness to something positive. Realize that it is the accumulated pressure of feelings that causes thoughts. So by freeing yourself from the painful feelings, it is actually possible to let go of thousand of thoughts associated with that feeling. In doing so, you may actually forget the event that caused you to have those thousands of thoughts. Don't ask yourself why you feel the way that you do, the mind will search for justifications. Let go of the thoughts and focus only on the feeling. Release the energy behind the feeling. The feelings you surrendered may come back. This is because there is more to be released. For years, you suppressed them, so don't criticize yourself and give up the process. Continue to surrender until you feel lighter and happier. Even in peace, learn to surrender that feeling so that you won't be attached to that outcome. Attachment to an outcome is another form of suffering through expectations.

Surrender is the only way to freedom!

The End, Never Ending Beginning

When was the last time you followed the movement of a wave from the ocean? It comes from an area in the ocean one does not know exactly from where, but at a certain point it raises itself up in the air, comes down crashing on the sand and retrieves back from where it came from. On and on, this process continues. So is your life, a continuous process of ever ending waves to ride on.

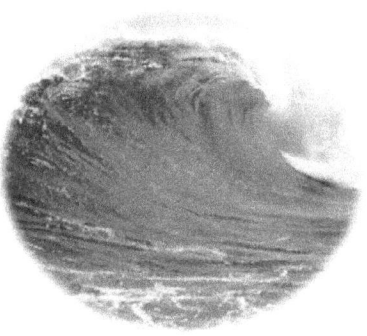

Let's suppose that you want to learn how to surf. Would you be able to do so if there wouldn't be any waves? Of course not! Following the same logic, is it possible that wanting to learn about life you are choosing to ride some waves once in a while? Watch a surfer and see what he does. He starts to learn by riding smaller waves. He expects to fall…that is part of the process. He gets back up on top of the wave. Once he becomes better at it, he will challenge himself and venture out to surf on top of bigger waves; in fact he welcomes the challenge, so he can perfect his skill. The bigger the wave, the greater the challenge, the greater the reward.

Watch him closely. He already knows that the key to his success is not to go against the current, but to merge with the flow of the wave and follow its movement.

Now, let's observe the process of your life. In a very similar way, you learn to master your skills by observing, practicing, falling, overcoming, and perfecting the challenges of your life. The greater the challenge, the greater the reward. Which reward, you may ask? Could it be something as simple as what the surfer experienced? The pure satisfaction of overcoming the challenges that were presented to you in this lifetime in order to perfect your skills at living at better life and evolve.

Is the surfer risking his life surfing? Sure he is! After all, there are sharks in the ocean. But, since he wants to learn to surf, he has to conquer his fears and accepts that it is part of the sport that he wants to learn. So, whether he is riding on top or falls, he does not concentrate on the dangers of surfing. His intention is to perfect his surfing without going against the current. Surrendering to the wave, the surfer's goal is to be taken to shore.

Can you surrender to your lives in the knowingness that you will make it safe to shore? Surrendering allows you to accept that there is a flow in the universe that is overseen by a force greater than yourself, greater than the majestic ocean. Yes, there will be storms, there will be calm, there will be small waves and bigger ones and that's all a part of it. If it would be calm all the time, how could you learn to surf?

When was the last time you walked by the ocean? Simply imagine yourself walking by the ocean. Close your eyes and see how it feels to be there. Can you imagine yourself being one with the waves of your life?

Let's just pretend that you are one of the waves crashing down on the sand, finally arriving at its destination. Where did you come from? Where did you start? What did you have to go through to get here? How long has been since you left? How was your journey? Did you become part of a hurricane or perhaps even more dramatic, a tsunami? Did people fear you or did you make them feel happy as you greet them gently, touching their feet.

Did you ever feel out of control when the storm took over your whole body and shaped you into a different form or did you simply surrender, knowing that your destiny was to be here one day? Simply arriving in serenity on a shore somewhere, where you could rest even for just one moment before being taken away for your next journey. Where are you going? Just a moment ago, you were greeting someone's feet and you just disappeared. Where are you? You lost your identity as you merged with the ocean.

Do you see the similarity of the wave with your own journey? Will you be able to peacefully surrender to your destiny resting for a moment before taking your eternal movement? Perhaps you could even lose your "self" and finally understand the meaning of your journey. Only then, could you gradually disappear along with the other waves as your companions and inseparably *together you would become ONE with the ocean.*

I hope you have enjoyed our odyssey together. This is the end of my book, but as you know me by now it is only the beginning. *Your beginning.* What do you desire to create in your life? And, most importantly, with which emotion? You always choose.

Which action will you take next? Yes, your life belongs to you but *"your life is not about you"* declares God to Neale Donald Walsch. When I read that simple sentence, something extraordinary becomes alive inside of me. That part of me that resonates with this simple truth that my life, my story resides in a very sacred way in your heart and soul. Then, I ask myself the same question, what do I desire to create? The desire to ignite in you a light, a force to heal your own life and go tell others about you. *Tell them that your story is not about you or I, but all of us together,* being One with the ocean of life. And, that together we can co-create a better world *by changing first the world that live inside each and everyone of us.*

You are Eternal! And so is your story forever written in your soul.

Appendix A

Feelings when your needs are not satisfied

AFRAID
apprehensive
dread
foreboding
frightened
mistrustful
panicked
petrified
scared
suspicious
terrified
wary
worried

ANNOYED
aggravated
dismayed
disgruntled
displeased
exasperated
frustrated
impatient
irritated
irked

ANGRY
enraged

CONFUSED
ambivalent
baffled
bewildered
dazed
hesitant
lost
mystified
perplexed
puzzled
torn

**DISCONNEC
TED**
alienated
aloof
apathetic
bored
cold
detached
distant
distracted
indifferent
numb
removed
uninterested
withdrawn

**EMBARRASS
ED**
ashamed
chagrined
flustered
guilty
mortified
self-conscious

FATIGUE
beat
burnt out
depleted
exhausted
lethargic
listless
sleepy
tired
weary
worn out

PAIN
agony
anguished
bereaved
devastated
grief

TENSE
anxious
cranky
distressed
distraught
edgy
fidgety
frazzled
irritable
jittery
nervous
overwhelmed
restless
stressed out

**VULNERABL
E**
fragile
guarded
helpless
insecure
leery
reserved
sensitive
shaky

furious
incensed
indignant
irate
livid
outraged

ANGRY
resentful

AVERSION
animosity
appalled
contempt
disgusted
dislike
hate
horrified
hostile
repulsed

DISQUIET
agitated
alarmed
discombobulate
d
disconcerted
disturbed
perturbed

DISQUIET
rattled
restless
shocked
startled
surprised
troubled
turbulent
turmoil
uncomfortable
uneasy
unnerved
unsettled
upset

heartbroken
hurt
lonely
miserable
regretful
remorseful

SAD
depressed
dejected
despair
despondent
disappointed
discouraged
disheartened
forlorn
gloomy
heavy hearted
hopeless
melancholy
unhappy
wretched

YEARNING
envious
jealous
longing
nostalgic
pining
wistful

Appendix B

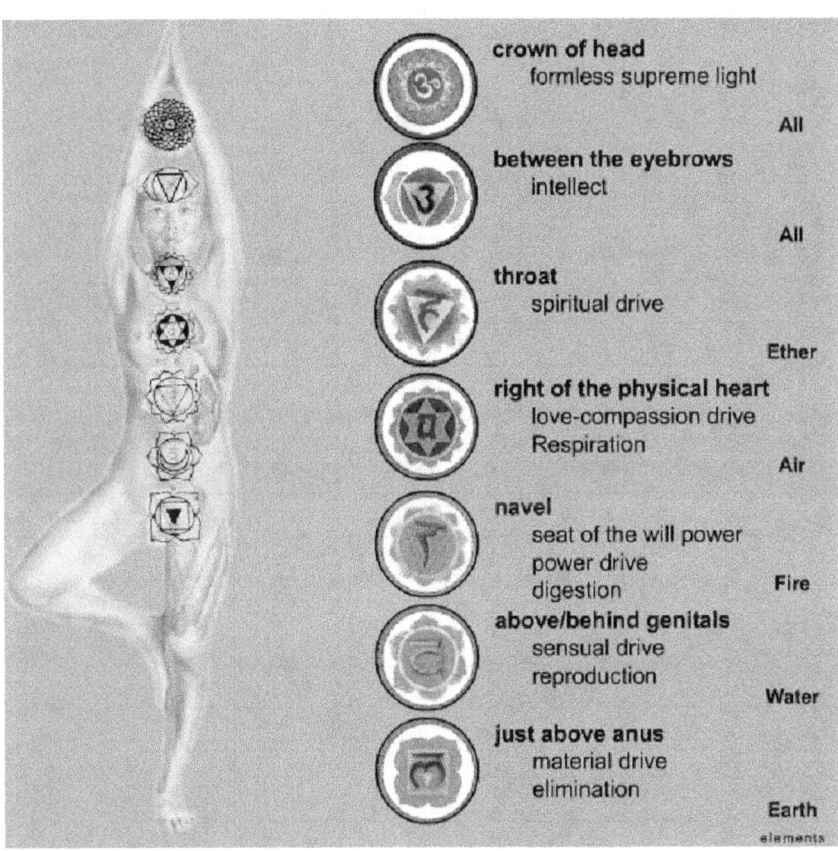

crown of head
  formless supreme light

All

between the eyebrows
  intellect

All

throat
  spiritual drive

Ether

right of the physical heart
  love-compassion drive
  Respiration

Air

navel
  seat of the will power
  power drive
  digestion

Fire

above/behind genitals
  sensual drive
  reproduction

Water

just above anus
  material drive
  elimination

Earth

elements

Appendix C

	Level	Scale (Log of)	Emotion	Process	Life-View
P O W E R	Enlightenment	700-1,000	Ineffable	Pure Consciousness	Is
	Peace	600	Bliss	Illumination	Perfect
	Joy	540	Serenity	Transfiguration	Complete
	Love	500	Reverence	Revelation	Benign
	Reason	400	Understanding	Abstraction	Meaningful
	Acceptance	350	Forgiveness	Transcendence	Harmonious
	Willingness	310	Optimism	Intention	Hopeful
	Neutrality	250	Trust	Release	Satisfactory
	Courage	200	Affirmation	Empowerment	Feasible
F O R C E	Pride	175	Dignity (Scorn)	Inflation	Demanding
	Anger	150	Hate	Aggression	Antagonistic
	Desire	125	Craving	Enslavement	Disappointing
	Fear	100	Anxiety	Withdrawal	Frightening
	Grief	75	Regret	Despondency	Tragic
	Apathy	50	Despire	Abdication	Hopeless
	Guilt	30	Blame	Destruction	Condemnation (Evil)
	Shame	20	Humiliation	Elimination	Miserable